I0696089

Dynamic 6

Packs

"Unlocking the Secrets to Sculpting Strong and Flexible Abs"

Jeremy Greeves

Copyright © 2023 by Jeremy Greeves

All rights reserved. No part of this publication may be reproduced, distributed, or transmitted in any form or by any means, including photocopying, recording, or other electronic or mechanical methods, without the prior written permission of the publisher, except in the case of brief quotations embodied in critical reviews and certain other noncommercial uses permitted by copyright law.

This book is intended for informational purposes only and is not meant to provide medical advice. The author and publisher are not responsible for any consequences that may arise from the use of this book.

TABLE OF CONTENTS

INTRODUCTION

Welcome to "Dynamic 6 Packs" – your ultimate guide to achieving and maintaining a strong, chiseled core. Whether you're an athlete, fitness enthusiast, or simply someone looking to enhance your physical prowess, this book is here to empower you on your journey to sculpting those coveted six-pack abs.

In a world where image and physical fitness are highly valued, having a well-defined midsection has become a symbol of strength, discipline, and aesthetic appeal. However, achieving a dynamic set of six-pack abs goes far beyond mere appearance. It signifies a deep level of core strength, stability, and overall fitness that can greatly enhance your performance in various sports, activities, and even daily life.

"Dynamic 6 Packs" dives deep into the intricate world of abdominal muscles, guiding you through the science, techniques, and exercises necessary to unleash the full potential of your core. This book is not just about crunches or sit-ups; it's about cultivating a comprehensive understanding of your abdominal anatomy and unlocking the secrets to dynamic, functional strength.

Within these pages, you'll explore the vital connection between proper nutrition and the development of a strong core. Discover the power of fueling your body with the right foods and supplements, enabling your abs to flourish and thrive.

But it doesn't stop there. This book will introduce you to a wide array of dynamic exercises specifically designed to target and challenge your abdominal muscles in innovative ways. From bodyweight movements to advanced resistance training techniques, you'll uncover a treasure trove of exercises that will push your core to its limits, increasing both strength and endurance.

Flexibility and mobility are equally crucial components of a truly dynamic core. Through expert guidance and effective stretching routines, you'll learn how to achieve and maintain optimal flexibility, enhancing your performance and reducing the risk of injuries.

Moreover, this book will delve into the world of advanced techniques, showing you how to take your core training to the next level. Unleash the power of high-intensity interval training (HIIT) and resistance exercises to sculpt your abs with precision, creating definition and symmetry.

Additionally, this book recognizes that different sports and activities demand specific core training approaches. You'll find tailored exercises and training plans for activities such as running, swimming, martial arts, and more, helping you excel in your chosen pursuits.

Prepare yourself for an enlightening journey through the core – not just as a destination for aesthetics but as a foundation of strength and resilience. By the end of the book, you will possess the knowledge, tools, and motivation needed to transform your core into a powerhouse of dynamic strength and vitality.

So, are you ready to embark on this transformative quest? Let's unlock the true potential of your abdominal muscles and set you on the path towards a strong, dynamic, and awe-inspiring six-pack. Let's dive in and embrace the incredible journey that lies ahead!

CHAPTER 1: ANATOMY OF THE ABDOMINAL MUSCLES

In this chapter, we will embark on an enlightening exploration of the intricate structure and functions of the muscles that make up the core. Understanding the anatomy of the abdominal muscles is crucial for anyone looking to develop a strong, dynamic set of six-pack abs.

We will delve into the different muscle groups that constitute the abs, such as the rectus abdominis, obliques, and transverse abdominis. You will gain a comprehensive understanding of their unique roles and how they work together synergistically to provide core stability and support.

Through detailed descriptions, diagrams, and illustrations, you will learn the specific attachments and actions of each muscle group. Discover how the rectus abdominis contributes to trunk flexion and plays a significant role in achieving those sought-after defined abs. Gain insight into the obliques, which are responsible for trunk rotation and

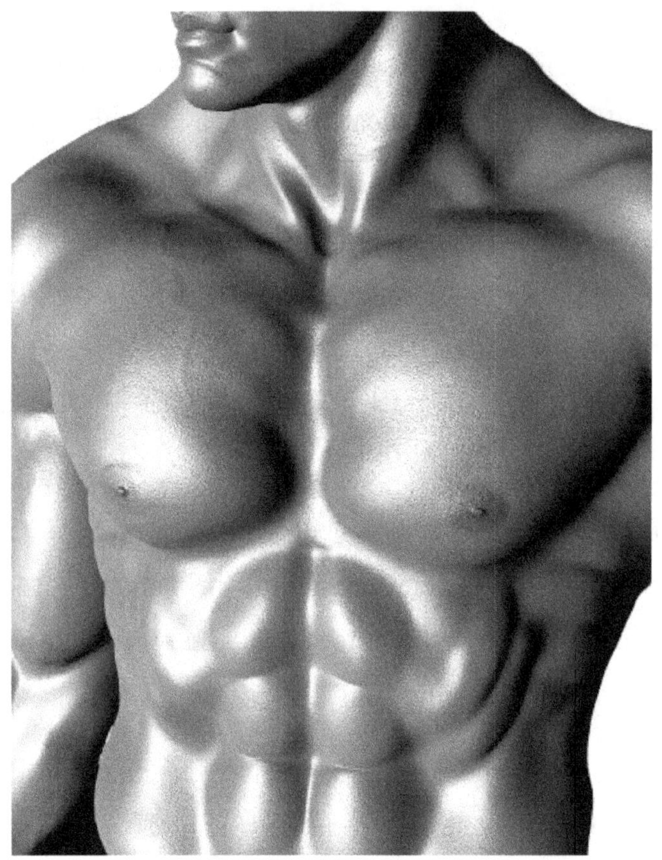

Picture of abdominal muscles with the upper body muscles

side-bending, and understand how they contribute to overall core strength.

Moreover, we will explore the deeper layers of the core, focusing on the transverse abdominis—a crucial muscle for core stability and spinal support. Understand the transverse abdominis' role in creating intra-abdominal pressure and its significance in maintaining proper form during exercises and daily movements.

By comprehending the intricacies of the abdominal muscles, you will not only enhance your knowledge but also refine your training approach. You will be able to target specific muscle groups effectively, ensuring balanced development and functional strength.

Throughout this chapter, we will also discuss common misconceptions and debunk myths surrounding abdominal training. By separating fact from fiction, you will gain a solid foundation of knowledge that will guide you towards intelligent and effective training methods.

Understanding the anatomy of the abdominal muscles is the first step towards unlocking the true potential of your core. It is the key that opens the door to developing a powerful, dynamic set of six-pack abs that goes beyond mere aesthetics. So, let's embark on this enlightening journey into the intricate world of the abdominal muscles and lay the foundation for a strong, functional, and awe-inspiring core.

Understanding The Different Muscle Groups That Make Up the Abs

Within your core lie various muscle groups, each with its own unique role and contribution to overall core strength and function. By understanding the different muscle groups that make up the abs, you will gain invaluable insights into how they work together harmoniously to provide stability, power, and fluid movement.

At the heart of your abdominal muscles is the rectus abdominis, commonly known as the "six-pack" muscle. This long, vertically-oriented muscle runs along the front of your abdomen, and its primary function is to flex the spine, bringing the ribcage closer to the pelvis.

On either side of the rectus abdominis, you will find the external obliques and internal obliques. These muscles wrap around your sides, forming a corset-like structure. The external obliques are responsible for rotating and bending the trunk, while the internal obliques assist in these movements and provide stability to the core.

Deep within your core lie the transverse abdominis muscles, which act as a natural girdle around your waist. These muscles provide crucial support and stability to the spine and pelvis, acting like a built-in weight belt that enhances core strength and protects against injuries.

In addition to these major muscle groups, the abdominal area also includes other supporting muscles, such as the serratus anterior, which assists in trunk rotation, and the pyramidalis, which aids in spinal flexion.

By unraveling the intricacies of each muscle group, you will gain a comprehensive understanding of how they work together synergistically to create a strong and dynamic core. With this knowledge, you will be equipped to target specific areas, customize your training, and maximize the effectiveness of your workouts.

So, let's dive deeper into the anatomy of the abdominal muscles and unlock the secrets behind their functions, interactions, and the extraordinary potential they hold for sculpting a powerful, dynamic core.

How Each Muscle Group Contributes to Core Stability and Movement

Here, we will explore the intricate relationship between the different muscle groups of the abdomen and their roles in maintaining stability and enabling fluid movement.

The rectus abdominis, often referred to as the "six-pack" muscle, plays a significant role in core stability and movement. Located at the front of the abdomen, it acts as a powerful flexor of the spine, allowing for movements such as crunches and sit-ups. By contracting and shortening, the rectus abdominis helps to bring the ribcage closer to the pelvis, creating flexion and contributing to trunk stabilization.

Moving to the sides, we encounter the external and internal obliques. These muscles wrap around the torso, forming diagonal layers that provide stability and facilitate various movements. The external obliques, positioned closer to the surface, assist in rotating and bending the trunk. They also work in conjunction with the internal obliques, which lie underneath, to produce lateral flexion and aid in rotational movements. Together, these muscles play a crucial role in generating rotational power and maintaining core stability during activities such as twisting, turning, and side-bending.

Deep within the core lies the transverse abdominis, often considered the body's natural corset. This muscle acts as a deep stabilizer, providing support and compressing the abdominal contents. Its horizontal orientation allows it to wrap around the waist like a belt, working in harmony with the other abdominal muscles to provide stability and protect the spine. The transverse abdominis is particularly vital for core stability during dynamic movements and acts as a foundation for generating power and transferring forces efficiently throughout the body.

In addition to the major muscle groups, other supporting muscles within the abdomen contribute to core stability and movement. The serratus anterior, located along the sides of the ribcage, assists in trunk rotation and protracts the scapulae, facilitating movements such as reaching and pushing. The pyramidalis, a small triangular muscle, aids in spinal flexion and provides additional support to the rectus abdominis.

By understanding how each muscle group contributes to core stability and movement, you will be better equipped to train your abs effectively and develop a well-rounded core. By targeting these muscles through specific exercises and movements, you can enhance their strength, coordination, and endurance, ultimately leading to improved performance, reduced risk of injury, and a more dynamic and functional core.

CHAPTER 2: NUTRITION FOR A STRONG CORE

In this chapter, we shift our focus from the physical aspects of core development to the vital role that nutrition plays in building and maintaining a strong core. While exercise and training are essential, without proper nutrition, your core's full potential may remain untapped.

We will delve into the symbiotic relationship between nutrition and core strength, uncovering the key nutrients and dietary strategies that fuel the growth and maintenance of your abdominal muscles.

One of the foundational elements of core nutrition is ensuring an adequate intake of high-quality protein. Protein serves as the building block for muscle tissue repair and growth. We will explore various sources of protein, both animal and plant-based, and provide guidance on determining the optimal protein intake for your individual needs.

In addition to protein, we will delve into the importance of carbohydrates for fueling your core workouts and replenishing glycogen stores. Carbohydrates provide the energy necessary to perform intense exercises, allowing you to push your core to its limits during training sessions.

Healthy fats also play a crucial role in core nutrition. We will discuss the different types of fats, such as monounsaturated fats and omega-3 fatty acids, that contribute to overall health, inflammation reduction, and optimal hormone function. Discover how incorporating the right types and amounts of fats into your diet can support core strength and enhance recovery.

While macronutrients form the foundation of core nutrition, we will also explore the significance of micronutrients, including vitamins, minerals, and antioxidants. These essential micronutrients aid in muscle function, repair, and overall health. We will identify key micronutrients that directly support core strength and discuss ways to incorporate them into your diet effectively.

Furthermore, hydration is often overlooked but critical for maintaining core health and performance. We will emphasize the importance of proper hydration and provide practical tips for ensuring adequate water intake throughout the day.

Lastly, we will address common dietary pitfalls and misconceptions surrounding core nutrition. Debunking myths and providing evidence-based recommendations, we aim to guide you towards making informed choices that support your core development goals.

By the end of this chapter, you will possess a comprehensive understanding of how nutrition directly impacts the strength, growth, and functionality of your core muscles. Armed with this knowledge, you will be empowered to make strategic dietary choices, optimizing your nutrition to fuel your core workouts, enhance recovery, and unlock the true potential of your abdominal muscles.

The Role of Diet in Building and Maintaining Abdominal Muscles

Diet plays a pivotal role in building and maintaining abdominal muscles. While exercise and training are crucial, it is through nutrition that the necessary building blocks and fuel for muscle growth and maintenance are provided. In this section, we will explore the vital role of diet in developing strong and defined abdominal muscles.

One of the key factors in building abdominal muscles is achieving a calorie balance that supports muscle growth. Consuming an appropriate number of calories ensures that your body has the energy it needs to build and repair muscle tissue. However, it is important to strike a balance between calorie intake and expenditure to avoid excess body fat that can obscure your abdominal definition. Understanding your individual caloric needs and finding the right balance is crucial.

Protein is a fundamental nutrient for muscle development, and it plays a particularly significant role in building abdominal muscles. Protein provides the necessary amino acids to repair and rebuild muscle tissue that undergoes stress during exercise. Including lean sources of protein, such as poultry, fish, eggs, dairy, legumes, and plant-based protein sources, in your diet is essential for providing the building blocks your body needs to create strong and well-defined abdominal muscles.

In addition to protein, carbohydrates are vital for fueling your workouts and providing energy for intense abdominal exercises. Carbohydrates are the body's primary source of fuel and are necessary for optimal performance during training sessions. Incorporating complex carbohydrates, such as whole grains, fruits, vegetables, and legumes, into your diet ensures a steady supply of energy for both your abdominal workouts and overall physical activity.

Healthy fats also play a crucial role in supporting abdominal muscle development. They provide essential fatty acids that contribute to hormone production and overall health. Including sources of healthy fats, such as avocados, nuts, seeds, olive oil, and fatty fish, in moderation, helps maintain proper hormone balance and supports the body's muscle-building processes.

Micronutrients, including vitamins and minerals, are often overlooked but are essential for optimal muscle function and recovery. They contribute to energy production, muscle contractions, and tissue repair. Consuming a varied diet that includes a wide range of fruits, vegetables, and whole foods ensures that you obtain the necessary micronutrients to support your abdominal muscle growth and maintenance.

Hydration is another critical factor in abdominal muscle development. Staying properly hydrated supports optimal muscle function, nutrient delivery, and waste removal. It is important to drink adequate water throughout the day to support your body's overall health and fitness.

While diet is crucial for building and maintaining abdominal muscles, it is important to note that spot reduction (losing fat specifically from the abdominal area) is not possible. To reveal your abdominal muscles and achieve a defined appearance, a combination of proper nutrition, regular exercise, and overall body fat reduction is necessary.

By understanding the role of diet in building and maintaining abdominal muscles, you can make informed choices about the foods you consume to support your fitness goals. A balanced diet that includes adequate protein, carbohydrates, healthy fats, micronutrients, and hydration will provide the foundation for strong, defined, and well-maintained abdominal muscles.

Recommended Foods and Supplements for Optimal Results

To achieve optimal results in building and maintaining abdominal muscles, incorporating specific foods and, if needed, supplements into your diet can be beneficial. Here are some recommended options:

Protein-rich foods: Include lean sources of protein such as chicken breast, turkey, fish (salmon, tuna), lean beef, eggs, Greek yogurt, cottage cheese, tofu, and legumes (lentils, chickpeas, black beans). These foods provide essential amino acids for muscle repair and growth.

Fruits and vegetables: Aim to include a variety of colorful fruits and vegetables in your diet. They are rich in vitamins, minerals, and antioxidants, which support overall health, muscle function, and recovery. Examples include berries, citrus fruits, leafy greens, broccoli, bell peppers, and sweet potatoes.

Whole grains: Choose complex carbohydrates like whole grains (oats, quinoa, brown rice), whole wheat bread, and whole wheat pasta. These provide sustained energy for workouts and help replenish glycogen stores in muscles.

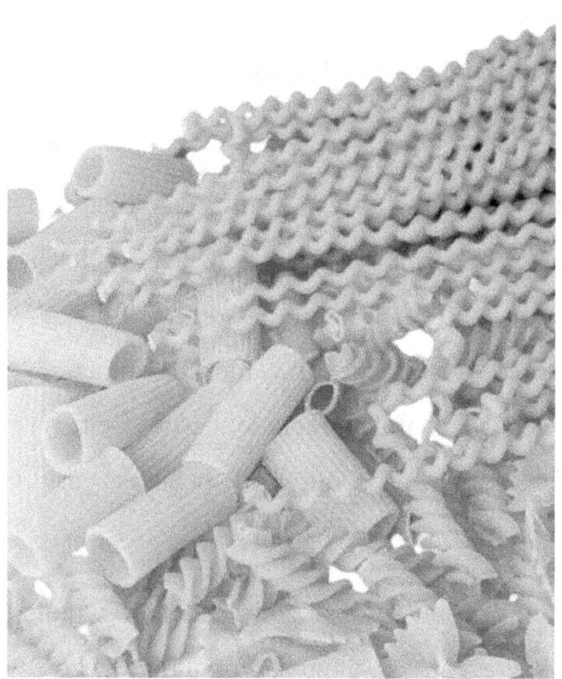

An Example of Whole Wheat Pasta

Healthy fats: Incorporate sources of healthy fats into your diet, such as avocados, nuts (almonds, walnuts), seeds (chia seeds, flaxseeds), olive oil, and fatty fish (salmon, mackerel). Healthy fats support hormone production, reduce inflammation, and aid in nutrient absorption.

Omega-3 fatty acids: If you don't consume enough fatty fish, consider omega-3 fatty acid supplements like fish oil or algae-based supplements. Omega-3s have anti-inflammatory properties and support muscle recovery and overall health.

Whey protein powder: Whey protein powder can be a convenient and effective way to increase protein intake and support muscle growth. It is quickly absorbed by the body and can be consumed as a post-workout shake or added to smoothies or recipes.

Creatine: Creatine monohydrate is a widely researched supplement that can enhance strength and muscle gains, including in the abdominal area. It can be taken as a supplement powder or found in small amounts in meat and fish.

Vitamin D: Adequate vitamin D levels are crucial for muscle function and overall health. Exposure to sunlight and consuming vitamin D-rich foods like fatty fish, fortified dairy products, and egg yolks can help, but consult a healthcare professional if considering supplementation.

Remember, while supplements can support your efforts, they should not replace a well-balanced diet. It's always best to consult with a healthcare professional or registered dietitian to determine your specific nutritional needs and to ensure any supplements align with your goals and health status.

CHAPTER 3: DYNAMIC EXERCISES FOR A POWERFUL CORE

In this section, we will explore a range of dynamic exercises specifically designed to strengthen and develop your core muscles. Unlike traditional static exercises, dynamic exercises involve movement, challenging your core to stabilize and generate force throughout various planes of motion. These exercises not only enhance core strength but also improve coordination, stability, and functional performance. Some of these exercises include:

Plank variations: Planks are a foundational exercise for core strength, and by adding dynamic elements, you can further intensify the challenge. Explore plank variations such as plank jacks, mountain climbers, and plank rotations to engage multiple muscle groups simultaneously and enhance core stability and endurance.

Medicine ball exercises: Incorporating a medicine ball into your workouts can add resistance and increase the demand on your core muscles. Exercises like medicine ball Russian twists, woodchoppers, and overhead slams engage the abdominal muscles, obliques, and even the lower back, improving overall core strength and power.

Stability ball exercises: Utilizing a stability ball can add instability, forcing your core to work harder to maintain balance and control. Exercises like stability ball rollouts, pikes, and knee tucks challenge your core muscles to stabilize and contract dynamically, leading to improved core strength and coordination.

Rotational exercises: Rotational movements engage the obliques and deep core muscles responsible for twisting and turning. Exercises like standing cable rotations, Russian twists with a weight plate, and bicycle crunches target these muscles, improving rotational power and functional core strength.

Dynamic planks and bridges: Elevate your core workouts with dynamic variations of planks and bridges. Exercises like walking planks, side plank hip dips, and glute bridges with leg lifts introduce movement and increase the challenge to your core muscles, enhancing stability, strength, and endurance.

Pilates and yoga-inspired moves: Pilates and yoga exercises emphasize core engagement and integration throughout various movements. Incorporate exercises like Pilates leg circles, boat pose, and yoga's downward dog to plank transitions to promote core strength, flexibility, and mind-body connection.

Explosive exercises: Plyometric exercises that involve explosive movements, such as medicine ball slams, standing broad jumps, and burpees, engage your core muscles in a dynamic and powerful manner. These exercises improve core stability, strength, and the ability to generate force rapidly.

Remember to focus on proper form and technique while performing dynamic core exercises. Gradually progress the intensity and difficulty of the exercises as your core strength improves. As always, consult with a fitness professional or trainer to ensure exercises are appropriate for your fitness level and to receive guidance on proper execution and modifications if needed.

By incorporating dynamic exercises into your core training routine, you will develop a powerful and resilient core that supports you in various athletic endeavors, functional movements, and everyday activities. The dynamic nature of these exercises enhances core functionality and prepares you for the dynamic challenges of real-life movements, contributing to improved overall fitness and performance.

Dynamic Warm-Up Exercises for The Abs

Dynamic warm-up exercises for the abs are an effective way to prepare your core muscles for a workout or physical activity. These exercises increase blood flow, activate the abdominal muscles, and improve flexibility and mobility. Here are some dynamic warm-up exercises specifically targeting the abs:

Standing Torso Twists: Stand with your feet shoulder-width apart, arms extended out to the sides. Rotate your torso from side to side, engaging your abs and obliques. Start with a slow and controlled movement, gradually increasing the speed and range of motion.

Cat-Cow Stretch: Start on your hands and knees in a tabletop position. Inhale and arch your back, dropping your belly towards the floor and lifting your head and tailbone. Exhale and round your back, pulling your belly button towards your spine and tucking your chin. Repeat this fluid motion, coordinating the movement with your breath.

Leg Swings: Stand next to a wall or sturdy object for support. Swing one leg forward and backward, maintaining a straight leg and engaging your core for stability. Repeat for several swings and then switch to the other leg. This exercise engages your abs and hip flexors while improving flexibility.

Standing Side Bends: Stand with your feet hip-width apart, arms relaxed by your sides. Reach one arm overhead and bend your torso to the side, feeling a stretch along the opposite side of your waist. Return to the starting position and repeat on the other side. Focus on engaging your oblique muscles as you perform the side bends.

Dynamic Plank Shoulder Taps: Start in a high plank position, with your hands directly under your shoulders and your body in a straight line. Lift one hand off the floor and tap the opposite shoulder, then place it back down and repeat on the other side. Engage your core to maintain stability and control throughout the movement.

Seated Knee Tucks: Sit on the floor with your knees bent, feet flat on the ground, and hands resting on the floor behind you for support. Lean back slightly, engaging your abs, and lift your feet off the ground. Bring your knees towards your chest, then extend your legs back out. Repeat this knee tuck motion, focusing on controlled and fluid movements.

Remember to perform these exercises in a controlled and smooth manner, gradually increasing the intensity as you warm up. It's important to listen to your body and modify or adjust any exercises as needed. Incorporating dynamic warm-up exercises for the abs will prepare your core muscles for the upcoming workout, enhance your performance, and reduce the risk of injury.

Core exercises using bodyweight and equipment

Core exercises can be effectively performed using just your bodyweight or with the assistance of various equipment. Incorporating both bodyweight and equipment-based exercises can provide a well-rounded and challenging core workout. Here are some examples of core exercises using both approaches:

Bodyweight Core Exercises

Plank: Assume a push-up position, resting on your forearms. Keep your body in a straight line from head to toe, engaging your core muscles. Hold the position for a set amount of time, focusing on maintaining proper form and breathing.

Mountain Climbers: Begin in a high plank position. Drive one knee towards your chest, then quickly switch legs in a running motion. Continue alternating legs in a controlled and fluid movement, engaging your core throughout.

Bicycle Crunches: Lie on your back with your knees bent and hands behind your head. Lift your shoulder blades off the ground and simultaneously bring one knee towards your chest while extending the other leg. Rotate your torso, touching your opposite elbow to the bent knee. Alternate sides in a pedaling motion, engaging your abs.

Russian Twists: Sit on the ground with your knees bent and feet lifted off the floor, balancing on your sit bones. Clasp your hands together in front of your chest and twist your torso from side to side, touching the ground beside your hips with your hands.

Equipment-Based Core Exercises

Swiss Ball Rollouts: Start in a kneeling position with your forearms resting on a Swiss ball. Roll the ball forward, extending your arms and allowing your body to move forward. Engage your core to control the movement and roll the ball back in towards your knees.

Cable Woodchoppers: Attach a cable or resistance band at chest height. Stand perpendicular to the cable or band, holding the handle with both hands. Pull the handle diagonally across your body, rotating your torso and engaging your core. Return to the starting position and repeat on the other side.

Medicine Ball Russian Twists: Sit on the floor with your knees bent and feet lifted off the ground, holding a medicine ball in front of your chest. Rotate your torso from side to side, tapping the medicine ball on the ground beside your hips. Keep your abs engaged throughout the movement.

Hanging Leg Raises: Find a pull-up bar or similar apparatus. Hang from the bar with your arms extended. Engage your core and lift your legs up towards your chest, keeping them straight. Slowly lower them back down without swinging, maintaining control.

By incorporating a combination of bodyweight exercises and equipment-based exercises, you can target your core from various angles and intensities.

Progressions for increasing difficulty and building endurance

Progressions are essential for increasing the difficulty of core exercises and building endurance over time. By gradually challenging your core muscles, you can improve strength, stability, and overall performance. Here are some progressions to consider:

Plank Progressions

High Plank to Low Plank: Begin in a high plank position, then lower down onto your forearms one arm at a time. Alternate between high plank and low plank for a specified number of repetitions or time.

Plank with Leg Lifts: While holding a plank position, lift one leg off the ground, focusing on maintaining a stable core and avoiding rotation. Alternate between legs for a set number of repetitions or time.

Plank with Arm Lifts: Similarly, while in a plank position, lift one arm off the ground, focusing on maintaining stability and avoiding excessive movement. Alternate between arms for a set number of repetitions or time.

Mountain Climbers Progressions

Slow and Controlled Mountain Climbers: Perform Mountain climbers at a slower pace, focusing on maintaining a stable core and avoiding excessive bouncing or momentum.

Cross-Body Mountain Climbers: As you bring your knees towards your chest during mountain climbers, aim to touch your opposite elbow to your knee, engaging your oblique muscles more intensely.

Russian Twist Progressions

Weighted Russian Twists: Hold a weight plate, dumbbell, or medicine ball in your hands while performing Russian twists to add resistance and increase the difficulty.

Feet Elevated Russian Twists: Elevate your feet off the ground, either by placing them on a stability ball or an elevated surface, to increase the challenge and engage your core muscles more intensely.

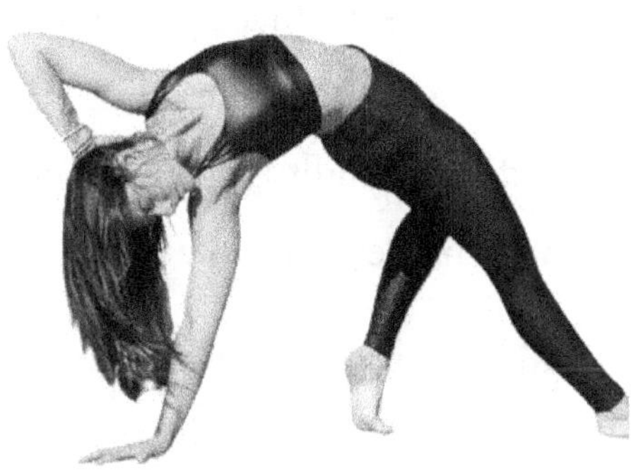

An Example of Russian Twist

Leg Raise Progressions

Hanging Knee Raises: Start with hanging knee raises, where you lift your knees towards your chest while hanging from a bar. Focus on maintaining control and avoiding excessive swinging.

Hanging Leg Raises: Once comfortable with knee raises, progress to straight leg raises, lifting your legs up towards the bar while keeping them straight. Control the movement and avoid swinging.

Exercise Ball Progressions

Plank on Exercise Ball: Place your forearms on an exercise ball instead of the floor while performing a plank. This adds instability, challenging your core muscles to work harder to maintain balance.

Stability Ball Rollouts: Assume a kneeling position with your hands on an exercise ball and roll the ball forward, extending your arms. Focus on maintaining a strong core and controlling the movement as you roll the ball back in.

Remember to always prioritize proper form and technique over speed or quantity. Gradually progress the difficulty and volume of your exercises as your core strength and endurance improve. Listen to your body, rest as needed.

CHAPTER 4: FLEXIBILITY AND MOBILITY FOR A HEALTHY CORE

Flexibility and mobility are crucial components of a healthy core. They contribute to proper posture, efficient movement, and reduced risk of injury. Here's a brief explanation of how flexibility and mobility impact core health:

Flexibility: Flexibility refers to the ability of your muscles and connective tissues to stretch and move through their full range of motion. Having good flexibility in the muscles surrounding the core, such as the hip flexors, hamstrings, and lower back, allows for optimal alignment and movement patterns.

Benefits for the Core: Improved flexibility in these muscles ensures that they can lengthen and contract efficiently during movements that involve the core, such as bending, twisting, and reaching. It helps prevent muscle imbalances and allows for proper engagement of the core muscles during exercises and everyday activities.

Mobility: Mobility refers to the ability to move a joint freely and actively, combining flexibility, joint stability, and motor control. It involves the coordination of muscles, tendons, ligaments, and joint structures.

Benefits for the Core: Adequate mobility in the spine, hips, and shoulders is essential for optimal core function. It allows for smooth and coordinated movement, facilitating proper activation and recruitment of the core muscles. Mobility also contributes to spinal stability, which is crucial for maintaining good posture and protecting the spine during various movements.

Stretching and mobility exercises to enhance range of motion

Stretching and mobility exercises are essential for enhancing range of motion and improving overall flexibility. By incorporating these exercises into your routine, you can increase joint mobility, reduce muscle tightness, and optimize your body's ability to move efficiently. Here are some stretching and mobility exercises to help enhance your range of motion:

Deep Squat: Stand with your feet shoulder-width apart, toes pointing slightly outward. Slowly lower your body into a deep squat, keeping your heels on the ground and your chest lifted. Use your elbows to gently push your knees outward, feeling a stretch in your hips, groin, and ankles. Hold the position for 30 seconds to 1 minute.

Standing Forward Bend: Stand with your feet hip-width apart and slowly bend forward from your hips, allowing your upper body to hang loosely. Let your arms hang towards the ground or reach for your shins, ankles, or the floor. Feel the stretch in your hamstrings, lower back, and calves. Hold the position for 30 seconds to 1 minute.

Butterfly Stretch: Sit on the floor with the soles of your feet together, knees out to the sides. Hold your feet or ankles, and gently press your knees down towards the floor. Feel the stretch in your inner thighs and hips. For a deeper stretch, gently lean forward while keeping your back straight. Hold for 30 seconds to 1 minute.

Thoracic Spine Rotation: Sit on the ground with your legs extended in front of you. Place your right hand behind your head and rotate your torso to the right, aiming to touch your left elbow to your right knee. Repeat on the other side. This exercise improves mobility and rotation in the thoracic spine.

Shoulder Circles: Stand tall with your feet shoulder-width apart. Extend your arms out to the sides at shoulder height. Make small circles with your shoulders, gradually increasing the size of the circles. Perform both forward and backward circles to mobilize the shoulder joints.

Cat-Cow Stretch: Start on your hands and knees in a tabletop position. Inhale as you arch your back, lifting your head and tailbone towards the ceiling (Cow pose). Exhale as you round your back, pulling your belly button towards your spine and tucking your chin (Cat pose). Move slowly and smoothly between the two positions, focusing on the movement and stretch in your spine.

Ankle Mobility Exercise: Sit on the edge of a chair or bench with your feet flat on the ground. Lift one foot off the ground and trace the alphabet in the air with your toes. This exercise helps improve ankle mobility and range of motion.

Remember to perform these exercises in a pain-free range of motion and never force a stretch.

Tips for preventing injury and maintaining flexibility

Preventing injuries and maintaining flexibility are important aspects of overall fitness and well-being. Here are some tips to help you in these areas:

Warm Up Properly: Always start your exercise sessions with a proper warm-up. Engage in light aerobic activities like jogging or jumping jacks to increase blood flow and raise your body temperature. Follow it up with dynamic stretching exercises that mimic the movements you'll be doing during your workout. This prepares your muscles, joints, and connective tissues for the upcoming activity and reduces the risk of injury.

Gradually Increase Intensity: When it comes to flexibility and physical activity, it's crucial to progress gradually. Avoid pushing your body beyond its limits too quickly. Increase the intensity, duration, or difficulty of your workouts gradually over time to allow your muscles and connective tissues to adapt and become more flexible.

Incorporate Regular Stretching: Make stretching a regular part of your routine. Engage in both static and dynamic stretching exercises to maintain and improve flexibility. Perform static stretches after workouts when your muscles are warm. Focus on major muscle groups, but don't neglect any specific areas that may be tight or prone to injury.

Focus on Proper Technique: When performing exercises or activities, ensure you use proper technique and form. This applies to weightlifting, sports, or any other physical activity. Incorrect form can place unnecessary stress on your muscles, joints, and ligaments, increasing the risk of injury. Seek guidance from qualified trainers or coaches to ensure you're using proper technique.

Listen to Your Body: Pay attention to your body's signals. If you experience pain, discomfort, or fatigue during an activity, take a break and rest. Pushing through pain can lead to further injury. Give yourself adequate time to recover and avoid overtraining, which can contribute to muscle imbalances and decreased flexibility.

Cross-Train: Engaging in a variety of activities and exercises can help prevent overuse injuries and promote overall flexibility. Incorporate different types of workouts such as strength training, cardiovascular exercises, and activities that challenge balance and coordination. This helps ensure that your body moves in various ways, promoting overall flexibility and reducing the risk of muscle imbalances.

Maintain a Balanced Lifestyle: A balanced lifestyle is essential for injury prevention and flexibility maintenance. Proper nutrition, hydration, and sufficient rest are vital for optimal recovery and tissue health. Additionally, incorporating stress-management techniques and getting enough sleep supports overall physical well-being.

Seek Professional Guidance: If you're unsure about proper techniques, training methods, or how to address specific flexibility concerns or injuries, don't hesitate to seek guidance from qualified professionals. Trainers, coaches, and physical therapists can provide personalized recommendations and assistance tailored to your needs.

CHAPTER 5: ADVANCED TECHNIQUES FOR SCULPTING THE ABS

Advanced techniques for sculpting the abs go beyond traditional exercises and challenge your core muscles in new ways. These techniques focus on intensity, variety, and progressive overload to help you achieve more defined and sculpted abs. Here are a few brief examples:

Resistance Training: Incorporate resistance training exercises specifically targeting the abdominal muscles, such as cable crunches, weighted Russian twists, or weighted decline sit-ups. Adding resistance through weights, resistance bands, or machines increases the difficulty and stimulates muscle growth, leading to more sculpted abs.

HIIT (High-Intensity Interval Training): Integrate high-intensity interval training into your workouts. This involves alternating between short bursts of intense exercises (such as mountain climbers, burpees, or planks) and brief rest periods. HIIT challenges your core muscles and helps burn excess fat, revealing the sculpted abs underneath.

Core Stability Exercises: Engage in advanced core stability exercises that challenge your balance and proprioception. Examples include plank variations on unstable surfaces like a stability ball or BOSU ball, side plank with leg raises, or plank jacks. These exercises enhance core strength, stability, and muscular endurance.

Pilates and Yoga: Incorporate Pilates and yoga routines that target the core muscles. These practices emphasize controlled movements, stability, and deep muscle activation. Exercises like Pilates leg circles, boat pose, or yoga boat pose (Navasana) engage the abs and contribute to sculpting the midsection.

Isometric Contractions: Include isometric exercises that require holding a static position to activate and strengthen the abdominal muscles. Examples include the plank hold, hollow body hold, or L-sit. Isometric contractions create tension in the muscles without joint movement and can lead to enhanced muscle definition.

We will shed more light on the first and second as these are known to build abs easily.

High-intensity interval training (HIIT) for the abs

High-intensity interval training (HIIT) for the abs is a game-changing approach to core training that will revolutionize the way you sculpt and strengthen your midsection. By incorporating HIIT into your abdominal workouts, you can maximize your results in less time while experiencing an exhilarating and challenging fitness regimen.

HIIT involves alternating between short bursts of intense exercise and brief recovery periods. This style of training not only boosts cardiovascular fitness but also elicits significant metabolic and muscular adaptations. When applied to abdominal exercises, HIIT can effectively target the entire core while elevating your heart rate, resulting in a dynamic and efficient workout.

In the chapter dedicated to HIIT for the abs, you will discover a wide range of high-intensity exercises specifically designed to engage and challenge your abdominal muscles. From explosive movements that activate the rectus abdominis to dynamic twists and rotational exercises that target the obliques, you will experience a diverse array of intense exercises that leave no muscle fiber untouched.

The beauty of HIIT lies in its versatility and adaptability to individual fitness levels. Whether you're a beginner or an experienced athlete, the exercises can be modified and progressed to suit your abilities. With each session, you'll witness your endurance and core strength soar to new heights.

But HIIT for the abs isn't just about burning calories and building strength. It also ignites your metabolic furnace, leading to increased fat burning long after your workout is complete. This metabolic boost is the result of the intense nature of HIIT, which stimulates your body's energy systems and promotes post-exercise oxygen consumption (EPOC). As a result, you'll continue to burn calories and fat even when you're at rest, accelerating your progress towards a lean and defined midsection.

In addition to providing a wealth of HIIT exercises, this chapter will guide you through proper form and technique, ensuring optimal results while minimizing the risk of injury. You'll also learn how to structure and customize your own HIIT workouts, allowing for flexibility and variety in your training routine.

So, get ready to embrace the intensity and power of HIIT for the abs. Experience the thrill of pushing your limits, breaking through plateaus, and unleashing the full potential of your core. Whether you're seeking a more defined six-pack or aiming to enhance your athletic performance, incorporating HIIT into your abdominal training will take you on a transformative journey towards a stronger, fitter, and more dynamic core.

Incorporating resistance training for maximum muscle growth

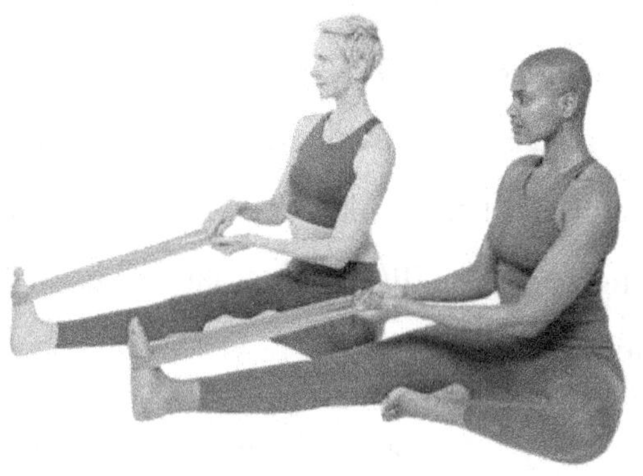

An Example of Resistance Training

Incorporating resistance training into your abdominal workouts is a game-changer when it comes to achieving maximum muscle growth and sculpting a strong, well-defined core. In this section, we will explore the benefits and strategies of incorporating resistance training specifically tailored for your abdominal muscles.

Resistance training involves working against an external force, such as weights, resistance bands, or even your bodyweight. While many people associate resistance training primarily with building muscle in the arms, legs, or back, it is equally effective for targeting and strengthening the abdominal muscles.

One of the key advantages of resistance training for the abs is that it allows for progressive overload. By gradually increasing the resistance or intensity of your workouts over time, you stimulate muscle growth and strength gains. This principle applies to your abdominal muscles as well, helping you develop a more defined, powerful core.

In our exploration of resistance training for the abs, we will introduce you to a variety of exercises and techniques that maximize muscle activation and growth. You will discover exercises such as weighted crunches, cable twists, and hanging leg raises, all designed to challenge your core muscles in new and demanding ways.

We will also discuss the importance of proper form and technique when incorporating resistance into your abdominal workouts. Emphasizing control and precision in your movements will ensure that you target the intended muscle groups effectively, reducing the risk of injury and optimizing your results.

Furthermore, we will explore different types of resistance equipment and tools that can enhance your abs training. From dumbbells and barbells to medicine balls and resistance bands, you will have a range of options to choose from based on your preferences and access to equipment.

Additionally, we will delve into strategies for periodization and progression in your resistance training routine. You will learn how to structure your workouts to continually challenge your muscles and prevent plateauing. By manipulating variables such as sets, reps, and weights, you will keep your abs workouts dynamic and stimulating, promoting continuous muscle growth and strength development.

Finally, we will discuss the importance of recovery and rest days in your resistance training regimen. Adequate rest is essential for muscle repair and growth, allowing your abdominal muscles to adapt to the demands placed upon them during your workouts.

By incorporating resistance training into your abs routine, you will unlock the potential for maximum muscle growth, strength, and definition. Whether you are aiming for a shredded six-pack or a stronger core for sports performance, resistance training is a vital component of your journey.

So, get ready to challenge your abdominal muscles in new and exciting ways as we explore the world of resistance training for maximum muscle growth. Let's elevate your core training to new heights and sculpt a powerful, dynamic set of abs that commands attention and showcases your dedication to strength and fitness.

Tips for targeting specific areas of the abs for a more defined look

To target specific areas of the abs for a more defined look, it's important to incorporate a combination of exercises that focus on the upper abs, lower abs, and obliques. Here are some tips to help you target these areas effectively:

Upper Abs

Crunches: Perform different variations of crunches, such as standard crunches, reverse crunches, or incline bench crunches. These exercises primarily target the upper portion of the rectus abdominis (six-pack muscles).

Cable Crunches: Utilize a cable machine to perform cable crunches. Attach a rope handle to the high pulley and kneel in front of it. Pull the cable down using your abs, bringing your chest toward your knees. This exercise provides constant resistance and can effectively target the upper abs.

Lower Abs

Leg Raises: Leg raises, including hanging leg raises, lying leg raises, or captain's chair leg raises, are effective for targeting the lower abs. Lift your legs while keeping them straight and lower them back down without touching the ground. Focus on using your lower abs to control the movement.

Reverse Crunches: Lie on your back with your knees bent and bring your knees towards your chest, lifting your hips off the ground. This exercise targets the lower abs and helps develop strength and definition in that area.

Obliques

Side Planks: Assume a side plank position, supporting your bodyweight on one forearm and the side of your foot. Keep your body in a straight line and engage your oblique muscles to stabilize. For an extra challenge, add hip dips or knee-to-elbow movements.

Russian Twists: Sit on the ground with your knees bent and feet lifted slightly off the floor. Twist your torso from side to side, touching the floor on each side. To increase the difficulty, hold a weight or medicine ball while performing the twists.

Full-Body Movements

Compound exercises that engage multiple muscle groups can indirectly target the abs while providing a calorie-burning effect for overall fat loss. Exercises like squats, deadlifts, push-ups, and overhead presses engage the core muscles for stability and can contribute to a more defined midsection.

Proper Nutrition

Remember that diet plays a crucial role in achieving a defined look. To reveal your abs, reduce overall body fat through a balanced and calorie-controlled diet. Focus on consuming nutrient-dense foods, adequate protein, healthy fats, and plenty of fruits and vegetables. Stay hydrated and avoid excessive consumption of sugary or processed foods.

CHAPTER 6: CORE TRAINING FOR SPECIFIC SPORTS AND ACTIVITIES

Core training for specific sports and activities involves tailoring exercises to enhance the specific movements and demands of the sport or activity.

Core exercises tailored to different sports, such as running, swimming, and martial arts

Here's a brief overview of how core training can be adapted for different sports and activities:

Running and Endurance Sports

Core Stability. Focus on exercises that improve core stability and endurance, such as planks, side planks, and bird dogs. These exercises help maintain proper posture and stability during long-distance running and repetitive movements.

Team Sports (e.g., Soccer, Basketball, Football)

Rotational Movements. Incorporate exercises that emphasize rotational movements, such as medicine ball twists or cable woodchops. These movements mimic the twisting and turning motions involved in these sports, improving power and agility.

Swimming

Anti-Rotation Exercises. Include exercises that resist rotation, such as Pallof presses or single-arm cable rows. These exercises help develop core stability and prevent excessive rotation during swimming strokes.

Martial Arts and Combat Sports

Dynamic Movements: Emphasize dynamic core exercises like medicine ball throws, rotational punches, or kicking movements. These exercises simulate the explosive and rapid movements required in martial arts, enhancing power and coordination.

Golf

Torso Rotation: Perform exercises that enhance rotational mobility and power, such as cable rotations or Russian twists with a golf club. These exercises strengthen the core muscles involved in generating torque and power during the golf swing.

Yoga and Pilates

Mind-Body Connection: Practice yoga or Pilates exercises that emphasize the mind-body connection and focus on core engagement, such as boat pose, plank variations, or the Pilates hundred. These exercises promote core strength, stability, and body awareness.

How to incorporate core training into your daily routine

Incorporating core training into your daily routine is a great way to improve core strength, stability, and overall fitness. Here are some tips on how to do it effectively:

Set Aside Dedicated Time: Allocate a specific time slot in your day dedicated to core training. This could be in the morning, during a lunch break, or in the evening. Consistency is key, so aim to train your core at least 2-3 times per week.

Start with a Warm-Up: Prior to engaging in core exercises, warm up your body with some light aerobic activity, such as jogging or jumping jacks. This helps increase blood flow, raise your body temperature, and prepare your muscles for the upcoming workout.

Mix and Match Exercises: Incorporate a variety of core exercises into your routine to target different muscle groups and keep things interesting. Include exercises like planks, crunches, Russian twists, bicycle crunches, leg raises, and mountain climbers. Aim for a balanced workout that engages the front, sides, and back of your core.

Progression and Challenge: As your core strength improves, gradually increase the difficulty or intensity of your exercises. This can be done by adding weights, increasing reps or sets, or incorporating more advanced variations of the exercises. Progression ensures continued growth and development of your core muscles.

Integrate Core Exercises into Workouts: Include core exercises as part of your overall workout routine. For example, add planks or bird dogs between sets of other exercises or perform core exercises as a circuit to maximize your training efficiency. This way, you're working on your core while also targeting other muscle groups.

Functional Movements: Incorporate functional movements that engage the core into your daily activities. Focus on maintaining proper posture and core engagement during tasks like lifting objects, carrying groceries, or performing household chores. This helps reinforce core strength and stability in real-life situations.

Balance and Stability Training: Integrate exercises that challenge your balance and stability, such as single-leg exercises or standing on an unstable surface (e.g., Bosu ball or balance board). These exercises engage the core muscles to maintain stability and improve overall core strength.

Be Mindful of Form and Technique: Pay attention to your form and technique during core exercises. Proper alignment and activation of the core muscles are essential for effectiveness and injury prevention. If needed, seek guidance from a qualified fitness professional to ensure you're performing exercises correctly.

Make it a Habit: Consistency is key when it comes to core training. Make it a habit by scheduling it into your daily routine and committing to regular sessions. Over time, it will become a natural part of your lifestyle.

CONCLUSION: THE ROAD TO A STRONG AND DYNAMIC CORE

Developing a strong and dynamic core is a journey that requires dedication, consistency, and a holistic approach to fitness. By following the principles outlined in this book, you have embarked on a path to transform your core strength, stability, and overall physical performance. Throughout the chapters, you have gained a deeper understanding of the anatomy of the abdominal muscles, the role of nutrition, dynamic exercises, flexibility, and targeted training for specific sports or activities.

Remember, building a strong core is not just about aesthetics but also about enhancing functional movement, preventing injuries, and improving overall fitness. As you progress on this road, keep in mind the following key takeaways:

Knowledge is Power: Understanding the different muscle groups that make up the abs, how they contribute to core stability and movement, and the role of nutrition in building and maintaining abdominal muscles is essential. Equip yourself with the knowledge to make informed decisions about your training and nutrition.

Consistency is Key: Incorporate core training into your daily routine and commit to regular workouts. Make it a habit and stay dedicated to your goals. Progress gradually, challenge yourself, and continually strive for improvement.

Balance and Variety: Incorporate a balanced mix of exercises targeting all areas of the core, including the upper and lower abs, obliques, and deep stabilizing muscles. Vary your exercises, intensity, and training methods to continuously challenge your core and avoid plateaus.

Listen to Your Body: Pay attention to your body's signals and adjust your training accordingly. Rest and recover when needed, and don't push through pain or discomfort. Prioritize proper form and technique to maximize the effectiveness of your workouts and reduce the risk of injury.

Holistic Approach: Remember that core training is just one component of overall fitness. Maintain a well-rounded fitness routine that includes cardiovascular exercise, strength training for other muscle groups, flexibility and mobility work, and a balanced diet. All of these factors contribute to a strong and dynamic core.

As you continue on your journey, stay motivated, track your progress, and celebrate your achievements along the way. With perseverance and determination, you have the potential to achieve a strong and dynamic core that will support you in all aspects of your active lifestyle. Embrace the challenges, enjoy the process, and revel in the transformative power of a strong core.

REFERENCES AND
FURTHER READING

Clark, M. A., Lucett, S. C., & Sutton, B. G. (2018). NASM essentials of personal fitness training. Jones & Bartlett Learning.

McGill, S. (2015). Ultimate back fitness and performance (6th ed.). Backfitpro Inc.

Contreras, B. (2013). Bodyweight strength training anatomy. Human Kinetics.

Helms, E. R., Fitschen, P. J., & Aragon, A. A. (2014). Evidence-based recommendations for natural bodybuilding contest preparation: Nutrition and supplementation. Journal of the International Society of Sports Nutrition, 11(1), 1-20.

Schoenfeld, B. J., Grgic, J., Ogborn, D., & Krieger, J. W. (2017). Strength and hypertrophy adaptations between low- versus high-load resistance training: A systematic review and meta-analysis. Journal of

Strength and Conditioning Research, 31(12), 3508-3523.

Anderson, K., & Behm, D. (2004). The impact of instability resistance training on balance and stability. Sports Medicine, 34(5), 293-304.

Hatfield, F. C. (2006). Fitness: The complete guide (8th ed.). International Sports Sciences Association.

Ebben, W. P., & Jensen, R. L. (2002). Electromyographic and kinetic analysis of traditional, chain, and elastic band squats. Journal of Strength and Conditioning Research, 16(4), 547-550.

Chaudhari, A. M., & Michaud, T. J. (2012). Exercise techniques for improving performance and reducing injury risk. In W. R. Frontera, D. L. Delisa, & J. J. Bockenek (Eds.), DeLisa's physical medicine and rehabilitation: Principles and practice (5th ed., pp. 1069-1082). Lippincott Williams & Wilkins.

American Council on Exercise. (2021). Exercise library. Retrieved from https://www.acefitness.org/education-and-resources/lifestyle/exercise-library/

Note: The references provided above are general sources on fitness and exercise. For more specific information on the topics covered in this book, such as nutrition, core training, and sport-specific training, it is recommended to refer to scientific journals, specialized books, or consult with certified fitness professionals or sports trainers.

www.ingramcontent.com/pod-product-compliance
Lightning Source LLC
Chambersburg PA
CBHW081957260726
48659CB00009BA/2961